Congratulations

For taking ACTION
And picking up this book!

ACTION is one of the greatest superpowers EVER!

You have taken the first step in a series of small steps, if taken daily for a sustained period of time, will UPLEVEL your life like never before!

The Superpower Practice is designed to help you achieve powerful results, in just 2-20 minutes a day.
Small daily habits can change your life, BIGTIME!

And the thing is, it's so SIMPLE!

Keeping it small, means keeping it going.
We have all tried the quick fix path.
It doesn't work because it doesn't last.
The goal is to have sustainable habits.
Small steps taken consistently,
create huge leaps forward,
effortlessly!

I hope you enjoy this book! It is meant to inspire and help guide you to your best life,
forever!

w/ Love,
Natalie

ISBN: 1502753227
ISBN-13: 978-1502753229

the
SUPERPOWER
PRACTICE

the **POWER** of simple daily action

the
SUPERPOWER
PRACTICE

Natalie Galyon

Here's to the crazy ones,
the misfits,
the rebels,
the troublemakers,
the round pegs in the square holes ...
the ones who see things differently –

they're not fond of rules, and they have no respect for the status quo. ... You can quote them, disagree with them, glorify or vilify them, but the only thing you can't do is ignore them because they change things. ... They push the human race forward, and while some may see them as the crazy ones, we see genius, because the people who are crazy enough to think that they can change the world, are the ones who do.

-Rob Siltanen for Apple

We can do anything we want to do if we stick with it long enough.

- Helen Keller

Success is 1% inspiration and 99% perspiration

-Thomas Edison

THE OVERVIEW

The SUPERPOWER PRACTICE OVERVIEW

The SUPERPOWER Practice is a simple guide to creating daily rituals that you LOVE to do and can seamlessly fit in to your busy life.

WHO THIS BOOK IS FOR

- For busy people looking to up-level their life for good, in just minutes a day
- For people who are willing to consistently put in at least 2 minutes a day
- For people who will do the work: small efforts, repeated day in and day out

WHO THIS BOOK IS NOT FOR

- People who are looking for a quick fix
- People who are not willing to put in the time and effort
- People who are not ready to up-level their current life

What if I told you that you already have the superpowers within you to create whatever you want?

We are already equipped with all that we need, we just have not been taught how to find and use our powers. We have ability to draw power from abundant sources of energy from within.

You have the POWER to create:

Anything you want!

You can harness the power from within, in just a few minutes each day!

It takes small steps to get big things done!

Replace the old habits with new simple daily habits and watch your life start move forward in big ways!

In fact, just minutes a day can shift your entire perspective, mood, and focus all day long.

When you find the practices that you love, they will become second nature, easy sustainable good habits you will have for the rest of your life.

THE MORNING is a good time to PRACTICE

Each morning we are born again.
What we do today is what matters most.
-Buddha

Why the Morning?

Each morning is a blank slate to create any kind of day we want.

You have a choice to see each morning as a gift.

What tone do you want to set for your day?

The morning practice gives you a reason to get out of bed. It gives you focus and starts your day with a positive mindset.

Starting with a few simple rituals is an easy way to begin a series of results that'll power you through your day.

This book is designed to give you a starting foundation with the intention to experiment with what works best for you.

HOW TO DO THE PRACTICE

The following pages are filled with fun simple daily action practices from 1 minute to 20 minutes each.

THE RULES:
1. For 21 days do at least 1 practice a day
2. Put in the time
3. Do the work
4. Small efforts repeated day in and day out create Big Results
5. After the 21 days create your own SUPERPOWER Practice by adding practices until you reach a good balance of 15-20 minutes each day
6. Mix and match
7. Change it up-Keep it fresh
8. Do your practice Daily

EXAMPLE SUPERPOWER PRACTICE:
- Wake up 6:30 AM
- Make some coffee
- Start the SUPERPOWER Practice
- MINI MEDITATION   5 minutes
- ACTION BOARD   2 minutes
- GET UP OFFA THAT THING   3 minutes
- CHUNK IT DOWN   3 minutes
- SUPERPOWER POSE   2 minutes

TOTAL TIME: **15 minutes**

THE SUPERPOWER PRACTICE PRINCIPLES

The following 10 principles will help keep you focused and moving forward

1. **GET CLEAR**- Ask yourself the following question *what do I really want?* Do not expect an answer right away just keep asking.
2. **NON-NEGOTIABLE**- make The Practice happen. Choose to make it a non-negotiable part of your day.
3. **STAY FLEXIBLE-** *An unbending tree is easily snapped.* To make it sustainable you must be flexible.
4. **MOVE**-make sure you are moving your body once a day.
5. **FOCUS ON YOUR BIG LIFE**- We need to have something larger. What is your Mission/Legacy?
6. **Keep your WILLPOWER reserves full**- Don't sweat the small stuff! Keeping the reserves full allows better daily choices.
7. **BUILD YOUR GRIT MUSCLE**- Grit is the sum of small efforts, repeated day in and day out. Persistence and Focus are the 2 key ingredients of a successful practice.
8. **WAKE UP EARLIER**- make time for the practice. Wake up 10 minutes earlier to get it in.
9. **MAINTAIN A SENSE OF WONDER**-keep a childlike view of the world.
10. **HAVE FUN!** - The most important part of the practice.

The SUPERPOWER DECLARATION

Read the following out loud to yourself in a mirror:
- I will keep moving forward each day no matter how small the step is
- I create or allow everything that happens to me
- My life is Non-Negotiable and I am here to LIVE IT!
- I choose to be Excellent
- I am responsible for the life I live
- I will be kind to myself

Accept the following:
- It will be hard at times
- You will fail, sometimes
- There will be setbacks
- There are always Obstacles
- Life is a marathon not a sprint
- Your energy level is not constant. Just do your best
- You will fall just get back up as soon as possible, every time
- Results may not show-keep moving!

THE CHALLENGE

Tell Me,
What Will You Do With Your One Wild & Precious
Life?
-Mary Oliver

1. I challenge you to make a pact with yourself, that you will give 21 days to the PRACTICE. You can do anything for 21 days.

2. Then, I **challenge** you to pick the practices that you like and create a daily ritual as little as 5 to 20 minutes a day. Choose what is doable for you and works with your schedule.

3. At the end of the 21-day Practice, I **challenge you** to contact me and tell me how your life has changed for the good because of *the SUPERPOWER PRACTICE!*

Okay, Lets do this!

_____
(SIGN HERE)

Do not judge me by my successes, judge me by how many times I fell down and got back up again.

-Nelson Mandela

Creating the
SUPERPOWER Practice

SUPERPOWER POSE

Act as if what you do makes a difference,
because it does. -William James

Superpowers

Confidence-Strength-Power-Unstoppable

Create your **Power Presence**. The Superpower Pose changes how you and others perceive you. It also has an immediate change in your body chemistry, the chemicals that make you feel good, powerful, and strong. Body language is a strong communication tool that tells you and others who you are. It opens you up to show less fear and more confidence. Strike a pose! Be strong and powerful all day long!

ACTION
Channel your best Wonder Woman pose

- Toes facing forward
- Hands on Hips
- Stick chest out
- Shoulder back
- Chin up
- Repeat a powerful mantra (silently or out loud) "I'm unstoppable, I'm powerful, I can do anything"
- Hold pose and repeat mantra for 1 minute

TIME: 1 minute

GET UP OFFA THAT THING

*Those who think they have no time for exercise will sooner
or later have to make time for illness.-Edward Stanley*

Superpowers

Strength-Confidence-Rocking Body-Inspiration

Get you blood flowing and boost your happy! Quick daily
exercise is one of the best ways to energize your day.
Making time for exercise provides some serious benefits
and you can do the following anywhere.

ACTION
Any exercise is good exercise. Get your bootie moving!

1. 20 jumping jacks
2. Jog in place 20 seconds
3. 20 jumping jacks
4. Butt kicks 20
5. 10 push-ups
6. 20 sit-ups
7. 10 push-ups
8. 20 sit-ups
9. 20 but kicks

TIME: 3 minutes

CHUNK IT DOWN

The secret of getting ahead is getting started. The secret to getting started is breaking your complex overwhelming tasks into small manageable tasks, starting on the first one.
- Mark Twain

Superpowers

Power-Confidence-Achievement

This is one of the most important practices in the book. *Chunking* is creating mini-goals each day. Daily mini goals help you feel a constant sense of achievement, which spills into all areas of your life. Start small and follow thorough.

ACTION
Start with a daily to do list of 4 mini-goals to achieve today.

- Pick your easiest one to do first. Moving through the list strengthens your willpower.
- DO this daily.
- If you do not get all goals done, move it to the next day's list.
- This small list done daily will move your life forward in big ways.
- BONUS: If you write the list the night before your subconscious will prep an overnight jumpstart for the day ahead.

TIME: 3-5 minutes

MIRROR MIRROR

It's not your job to like me, it's mine.
-Byron Katie

Superpowers
Self Love-Confidence-Compassion

What do you say to yourself when you look in the mirror?

A few positive words each day can lift you up to the next level. Unleash that inner DIVA with Mantras that light you up inside! This is an action of self Love with POWER! You are your best friend and support, so treat yourself with compassion and LOVE.

ACTION
Use the example mantras below or find mantras that light you up!

- Look yourself in the mirror.
- Take a couple of deep breaths.
- Focus on the woman staring back at you.
- Tell her that this is a safe place with no judgment.
- Smile at her.

Repeat, for 1 Minute, the following Mantras:
(Or replace with mantras that energize you)

- Today I create my OWN Sunshine
- Be the reason someone SMILES today
- I am a Beautiful work in progress
- It's a good day to have a GOOD day
- I may not be perfect but parts of me are Pretty Awesome
- I am LOVED
- It might take a day, it might take a year but it WILL happen
- I am my OWN unique self – special, creative and wonderful.
- I make SH*T happen
- I am not a tree- so get MOVING!
- Be the type of person I want to meet
- I Focus on the GOOD

TIME: 2 minutes

BREATHE

Alive or just breathing?
-Unknown

Superpowers

Laser Focus-Relaxation-Anxiety Buster

Deep breathing is one of the best ways to lower stress in the body by sending a message to your brain to calm down and relax. This simple Breathing practice is an essential tool for wellness and can be done anywhere, anytime.

ACTION

Controlled breathing helps with anxiety, stress, focus, sleep, and tension.

1. Sit in a comfortable position
2. Exhale completely through your mouth
3. Close your mouth and inhale quietly through your nose for 4 seconds. Hold for 6 seconds
4. Exhale completely through your mouth to a count of 7
5. Repeat 3 more times

TIME: 2 minutes

PLAY

Immature is a word that boring people use to describe fun people.- Will Ferrell

Superpowers
Joy-Youth-Happiness

"I wish I had worked less and played more"...
Don't let this phrase come from your lips, EVER!

WHAT IS PLAY?

Play is what it feels to be alive. Play is what we remember on our deathbed. Physical Activity is the most basic form of play. Play is: movies, art, music, silliness, games, and laughter.

ACTION
Think back to how you played as a child.
What did you play?
How did you feel? Alive, carefree, happy.
How could you play today? Take at least 5 minutes for play today.

- skipping
- laughing
- a short walk
- bike riding
- hiking
- games with your children or furry babies

- stand up comedy night
- camping
- cloud gazing while lying in the grass
- swimming
- learning something new
- building a sand castle
- painting

Time: 5+minutes

MINI MEDITATION

The quieter you become
the more you can hear.-Ram Dass

Superpowers
Stress Reliever-Clarity-Calmness

Life can be busy and hectic. Meditation is good for memory, stress and clarity, but most of us do not have the time or attention spans to sit for long periods of time. All it takes is 5 minutes for this mini mental boost!

Benefits
- Focus
- Mental clarity
- Good mood
- Calmness
- Relaxation

ACTION
Take time each day, or when you need to re-center, to practice you Mini Meditation.

Find a piece a music that is relaxing and is under 5 minutes long. Look for something that does not have lyrics and keeps your mind peaceful, such as classical guitar, meditation music, or Native American music.
- Find in a quiet comfortable space
- Relax into a comfortable siting position
- Start the music (wear headphones if you have

noise distractions)
- Close your eyes
- Focus on your breath and quiet the mind
- Focus on relaxing and breathing until the song is over

TIME: 3-5 minutes

DO WHAT SCARES YOU

Do you want to see something REALLY scary?
- Dan Aykroyd, The Twilight Zone Movie

Superpowers
Confidence-Unstoppable-Fearless

So, it's easier to not meet new people, not step on the scale, not go to the gym, not quit your job, not say I love you, continue doing the same things day in, day out. Do one thing a day that you fear. You will soon learn to be comfortable with the uncomfortable. As you progress, your goals and life dreams look less scary and become possible. What are you afraid of? OK go do it!

ACTION
1. Do one thing every day that you fear
2. Ask yourself, *what is the worst that could happen*?
3. Think about it, accept it and go do it.

Some examples:
- Try a new restaurant solo
- Going to a public place to work out
- Smiling at a complete stranger
- Learning something new
- Meeting new people

TIME: 1-5 minutes to decide/plan

MAKE MY DAY

No act of kindness, no matter how small, is ever wasted. –Aesop

Superpowers
Kindness-Love-Empathy

A DAYMAKER:

A person who performs acts of kindness with the intention of making the world a better place. One of the greatest gifts you can bestow upon another and yourself is to give kindness without the expectation of something in return.

ACTION
Plan it out or be spontaneous, just make someone's day!

- Tweet or Facebook message a genuine compliment to three people right now
- Let people merge in traffic today
- Make plans with that person you've been putting off seeing
- Purchase some extra dog or cat food and drop it off at an animal shelter
- When you hear that negative, discouraging voice in your head, be kind to yourself and remember "You are a beautiful work in progress"
- Say thank you to a janitor
- Give away stuff for free on Craigslist
- Smile at someone on the street, just because

- While you're out, compliment a parent on how well-behaved their child is
- Let someone that looks in a hurry ahead of you in line

TIME: 1+minute

SWAGGER
(aka swagga)

Some folks look at me and see a certain swagger, which in Texas is called WALKING. -"W"

Superpowers
Confidence-Calm-Cool

Swagger is person's style- they way they walk, talk, dress. Swagger is to move with confidence, sophistication and to be you. Swagger gives an aura of comfortableness, coolness, and togetherness.

ACTION

Be aware of how you carry yourself today. Do you carry yourself the same in different situations?

Try the following as you go about your day.

STAND TALL. -Height communicates stature & authority. Watch others and how they carry themselves. Become aware of how you carry yourself.

WALK WITH PURPOSE. When you walk down the street, don't slouch or hesitate. Hold your head up and know that you belong wherever you are!

RADIATE YOUR STYLE-. You are what you *wear*! Feeling

comfortable in your own skin radiates magnetism. Wear what makes you feel powerful confident, and sexy. Get dressed with purpose. Experiment and pay attention to how you feel wearing different garments. Not sure where to started? Get a personal shopper or online stylist. Many stores offer this service in person or online.

SMILE- Smile with your eyes and tone of voice. Smiling while you talk changes the energy and tone of your voice. Positive energy communicates self-love and inner confidence and can change the energy of the person you are communicating with.

TIME: 1+minute

LOVE FEST

Superpowers
Pain Reliever-Mood & Immunity Booster

A big bear hug, a cuddle with your dog, a quiet nap on the sofa with you children. Giving some lovin' to your pets, partner or children is the ultimate mind-body medicine.

From lowering blood pressure and heart rate to increasing immune function and relieving pain, cuddle time makes you healthier & happier. So cuddling with your dog might be the way to a happier, calmer you.

ACTION

Create a small moment each day to do some cuddling with you pet, partner or children.

TIME: 5 minutes

MODEL YOUR MENTOR

Be so good they can't ignore you.
-Steve Martin

Superpowers
Shape Shifter-Path Finder

Who is living your BIG LIFE?
Do what they do. Act how they act.

What do you want? A fit and healthy body, to be your own boss, swim the English Channel? Want to achieve what you want in a shorter timeframe, then seek out people who are living the life that you want and learn from them, fast. What are their daily habits and mindsets?

ACTION
Model someone who is achieving what you want.

- Do your research of at least 3 people doing what you would like to do.
- Reach out to them via, email, website, or Facebook. Ask them questions. Take them to lunch. Replicate their energy. They have a set of habits that are already working. They have written books, given ted talks, have podcasts, and blogs.

TIME: 5-20 minutes

WHAT'S YOUR STORY?

Owning our story and loving our selves through that process, is the bravest thing we will ever do.
- Brene Brown

Superpowers

Time Travel- Future Teller-Imagination

Take a moment and imagine it's toward the later years of your life. You have taken a moment as your future self to look back at your life. You can see yourself and your dreams as a child, as a teenager, young adult and as who you are now.

When you look back, are you living in alignment with what your dreams were as your younger self?

Maybe you have new dreams?

Are you happy when you look back?

What things do you wish you had done?

What kind of person do you wish you would have been?

ACTION
Now is the time to make things happen! Spend 5 minutes and write a super short story on the life you would love to live- Write it as your future self looking back on the BEST

life you can imagine. You can do or be anything. Write it as if you are living it now and about who you want to be and how you want to live life. Read it to yourself every morning.

Time: 5 minutes

WHY?

Words may inspire, but only action creates change. Most of us live our lives by accident – we live life as it happens. Fulfillment comes when we live our lives on purpose. -Simon Sinek

Superpowers
Clarity-Purpose

Time to get CLEAR! Most of us are on autopilot and drift through life because we have a vague sense of where we are going and why. Getting clear allows you to focus your energy on what matters. Knowing WHAT and WHY, you take more risks and keep moving forward in spite of all bumps in the road.

ACTION

Ask yourself the following questions. Do not expect an answer right away. Just ask and let it go. Repeat each day and observe what comes up. Clarity will come when you least expect it.

- What are you good at?
- What makes you come alive?
- What problems do you really enjoy solving?
- What will be your legacy?

TIME: 1 minute

MOVE!

Movement is a medicine for creating change in a person's
physical, emotional, and mental states.
-Carol Welch

Superpowers
Fitness-Strength-Optimism-Joy

Make daily **MOVEMENT** a non negotiable!

Exercise is the single most POWERFUL tool you have to optimize your life. Just 20 minutes a day can boost energy, strength, mood and brainpower. Walking for 20 minutes clears you head, upgrades your mood, and releases the good chemicals that promote optimism and joy!

ACTION
Make it your mission to find daily movement you love to do for at least 20 minutes day. Take a couple of minutes to brainstorm on as many different ways to get moving. Try them out and do the ones you love. Repeat 5-7 days a week

Dancing-Walking-Trampoline-Sprinting-Workout DVD-Yoga-Cycling-Zumba-Spin-Hula Hooping-Skipping-Hiking-Swimming

TIME: 20 minutes

THE IMPOSSIBLE

It's always impossible until it's done.
- Nelson Mandela

Superpowers

Confidence-Strength-Courage

Live a life of meaning and adventure by changing the impossible to I'm POSSIBLE!

DO...The things that people say can't be done.

DO...The things you never dreamed you'd be able to do.

Do...The things others said you'd never be able to do.

ACTION

Decide to Do Something!

What are 3 things that you think you can't do?

- Fear of Public speaking? - Join toastmasters or an Improv class
- Not a strong swimmer? - Take a lesson at your local YMCA
- Want to make 6 figure income- Find a business coach (student coaches are very low cost)

If you don't know how, find someone who does. There is always a way!

TIME: 2+minutes

HOLIDAY ROAD

This is no longer a Vacation. It's a quest. It's a quest for fun.
- Clark Griswold, Vacation

Superpowers

Excitement-Enthusiasm-Energy

Daydream and plan your next EPIC vacation. Travel has the potential to re-energize, and refocus our lives. Imagine feeling ready to take on the world again. Time to step out your comfort zone and push the limits. Try something new!

ACTION
Start planning now. Just a couple of minutes a day of planning your vacay will lift you up and open your mind to new possibilities.

- Create a Bookmark folder on your computer for your Vacation
- Google at least 1 idea a day
- Bookmark the webpage or copy an image that excites you and place in the folder

Fun Examples
- Yoga Retreat in Bali
- Month long hike on the Colorado Trail
- Week long surf camp in Costa Rica
- Helping the homeless dogs in Detroit
- Relax on a island bungalow in the Maldives

TIME: 5 minutes

POWER QUESTIONS

The question isn't who is going to let me; it's who is going to stop me.
-Ayn Rand

Superpowers
Purpose-Clarity-Flame Maker

Power questions are queries into our inner realm that may not evoke immediate answers. Just ask the question and then move on. We ask ourselves questions to gain clarity, inspire action, and discover who we are on a deeper level.

ACTION

If you really want to create a shift in your life success, make these power questions part of your daily ritual. Challenge yourself to find 5 power questions or use the examples below.

- What is possible?
- What if it works out exactly as you want it to?
- What does fun mean to you?
- How would you behave if you were the best in the world at what you do?
- Am I raising my standards?
- If you could do anything you wanted, what would you do?
- When you are ninety-five years old, what will you want to say about your life?
- How does this relate to your life purpose?

- In the bigger scheme of things, how important is this?
- So what?
- What is stopping you?
- If you had your choice, what would you do?
- What will happen if you do, and what will happen if you don't?

TIME: 1-3 minutes

CREATIVE BEAST

Think left and think right and think low and think high. Oh,
the thinks you can think up only if you try.
-Dr. Seuss

Superpowers
Creativity –Clarity

Removing clutter from your mind gives rise to your creativity!

In the morning, while your brain is still waking up, is a perfect time to get a pen and paper and start writing. About anything in fact, just let it flow. No rules just move the pen from left to right. This practice will clear your mind of all the stuff that gets in the way.

ACTION

- Get pen and notebook
- Start writing *stream of consciousness* style
- Fill up 1 page
- Your ideas and thoughts are now unleashed

TIME: 3-5 Minutes

ACTION BOARD *UPGRADED*

You can't be what you can't see.
-Miss Representation

Superpowers

Hope-Energy-Zest-Motivation

Put away your scissors, glue, poster board and magazines and UPGRADE to a **Virtual** Action board using your computer. Action Boards allow you to better visualize the small steps you need to take by seeing what you want every day.

Think of it as a map of your future that will inspire and help you on a daily basis, a daily reminder of what you want. It's that simple. The images will stimulate and help your mind remember what you want.

ACTION

Brainstorm What Moves You:

- Exercise, travel, dancing, cooking
- Become financially free, make $100,000
- RV, designer purse, iPad
- Adventure Travel to Bali, Take a Surfing Vacation, Hike the Continental Divide
- People Who Inspire You -Authors, Actors, Historical Figures, Mentors

- **PIN IT!** Make a board on Pintrest specifically for the vision you are working on. Then go searching and pinning from your brainstorming ideas.

- Once you have set up you Pintrest page, take 5 minutes each day to look at the images you have collected on Pintrest and add 1 new image per day.

TIME: 3-5 Minutes

microYOGA

Remember that your natural state is JOY.
- Wayne Dyer

Superpowers
Strength-Energy-Flexibility

YOGA CAN REALIGN YOUR MIND, YOUR BODY, AND
YOUR SPIRIT. ALSO YOGA BUILDS STRENGTH AND
INCREASES YOUR FLEXIBILITY.

MOST OF US DO NOT HAVE TIME TO DRIVE TO CLASS,
SPEND AN HOUR IN CLASS, THEN DRIVE HOME.
THIS SHORT MINI YOGA PRACTICE IS DESIGNED TO FIT
INTO MOST BUSY SCHEDULES.

ACTION
Try these mini-yoga poses anywhere to get stronger and
more flexible in minutes.

MOUNTAIN POSE
- Stand tall with feet together, shoulders relaxed,
  weight evenly distributed through your feet, arms
  at sides. Take a deep breath and raise your hands
  overhead, palms facing each other with arms
  straight. Reach up toward the sky with your
  fingertips.

Hold for 5 breaths

DOWNWARD DOG
- Start on all fours with hands directly under shoulders, knees under hips.
- Walk hands a few inches forward and spread fingers wide, pressing palms into mat. Curl toes under and slowly press hips toward ceiling, bringing your body into an inverted V, pressing shoulders away from ears. Feet should be hip-width apart, knees slightly bent.

Hold for 3 breaths

WARRIOR
- Stand with legs 3 to 4 feet apart, turning right foot out 90 degrees and left foot in slightly.
- Bring your hands to your hips and relax your shoulders, then extend arms out to the sides, palms down. Bend right knee 90 degrees, keeping knee over ankle; gaze out over right hand.

Stay for 1 minute

CHILDS POSE
- Sit up comfortably on your heels.
- Roll your torso forward, bringing your forehead to rest on the floor in front of you. Lower your chest as close to your knees as you comfortably can, extending your arms in front of you.

Hold the pose and breathe for 10 breaths

TRIANGLE POSE

- Extend arms out to sides, and then bend over your right leg.

- Stand with feet about 3 feet apart, toes on your right foot turned out to 90 degrees, left foot to 45 degrees.

- Allow your right hand to touch the floor or rest on your right leg below or above the knee, and extend the fingertips of your left hand toward the ceiling.

- Turn your gaze toward the ceiling

Hold for 5 breaths

Stand and repeat on opposite side

BRIDGE POSE

- Lie on back on floor with knees bent and directly over heels.
- Place arms at sides, palms down. Exhale, and then press feet into floor as you lift hips.
- Clasp hands under lower back and press arms down, lifting hips until thighs are parallel to floor, bringing chest toward chin.

Hold for 1 minute

Repeat the set 3 times

TIME: 9 minutes

FIND YOUR STRONG

A RIVER CUTS THROUGH ROCK, NOT BECAUSE OF ITS POWER,
BUT BECAUSE OF ITS PERSISTENCE.
-JIM WATKINS

Superpowers
Greatness-Higher Purpose

Your Strong = your BIG THING!

You wake up and notice its still dark outside. What time is it? Early...your mind starts to imagine your day ahead. You are so happy to be awake because you cannot wait to start the new day! You love your life and jump out of bed ready to take it on! Your energy is overflowing, all of this coming from deep inside your body. You love of being alive and knowing why you are here. You have a greater purpose and you are unstoppable!

So, What wakes you up in the morning?

What is alive in you?

What makes you JUMP OUT OF BED?

WE EXIST ON THIS EARTH FOR SOME UNDETERMINED PERIOD OF TIME AND THE IMPORTANT THINGS GIVE OUR LIVES MEANING AND HAPPINESS.

WHAT ARE THE IMPORTANT THINGS?

NONE OF US KNOW EXACTLY HOW WE FEEL ABOUT
SOMETHING UNTIL WE ACTUALLY DO SOMETHING.

ACTION

- PUT IN THE TIME AND WORK AND DO THE
  SMALL PRACTICES IN THIS BOOK DAILY AND
  YOUR **BIG THING** WILL RISE TO THE SURFACE!

TIME: FOREVER

MORE
POWERFUL
STUFF

- **BONUS** MINI NUTRITION PRACTICE
- ABOUT THE AUTHOR
- GET IN TOUCH

The Big Ass Salad (BAS)

Doctor says to patient: Stop eating your veggies. I can't seem to find anything wrong with you.

Superpowers
Radiance-Energy-Longevity

The BAS: The EASY and yummy way to get tons of veggies into you daily diet.

You have heard a million times, eat more veggies and fruit, and not much has changed over the years. So, are you taking this advice into daily practice? Chopping the salad into small pieces, allows you to pack in a ton of veggies without realizing it. You can chop with a knife but the real secret is the OXO salad chopper (no affiliation, just love it!). The OXO makes the BAS easy and fun.

One of the best things about eating a big ass salad is it keeps you full and satisfied, a huge step in maintaining or losing weight.

ACTION
Replace 1 meal daily with a BAS

What you need:
- OXO chopper (or chop with knife)
- 4 cups of greens (your choice-experiment)
- 8-10 cherry tomatoes

- Fist size of chicken (6 oz.) or any lean protein
- Cucumber
- Colorful peppers
- 2-3 Tbsp. EVOO based dressing
- 1-2 oz. cheese for topping (optional)

Place all veggies and protein into the chopper bowl and chop away. Add the salad dressing and top with cheese.

Make this a daily NON-NEGOTIABLE.
Go to www.gritstrong.com for more salad ideas.

TIME: 5 Minutes daily

EAT REAL FOOD

Low Sugar, High Fiber. That's the only diet that you need.
It's called eat real food.
-Robert Lustig, MD and author, Sugar the bitter truth

Superpowers

Radiance-Energy-Longevity

What do most of the successful diets, Paleo, Atkins, Mediterranean, South Beach, have in common? Low Sugar, High Fiber. When foods are processed, sugar is added to make it taste good and fiber is taken out for longer shelf life. One of the most important things you can do for your health is to decide to cut down or eliminate processed foods.

ACTION
- Eat real, whole foods
- Shop in the perimeter of the store. The stuff in the middle is mostly processed
- Look for foods with one ingredient
- Drink more water
- Avoid soda, sports drinks, juice
- Read labels- if you can't pronounce an ingredient, don't eat it

TIME: Daily

ABOUT THE AUTHOR

This book is a result of overcoming the struggle with weight and the fat free craze 80's-90's. Both which led to a becoming a master of self inflicted body shaming. The journey of losing 100lbs has sparked a passion for health and wellness
and an overwhelming drive to help others feel comfortable in their own skin.
I want to inspire and help guide women to learn to love their body and upgrade their life.
My **BIG THING** is helping rid the world of processed foods and teaching others how to be comfortable & confident with their bodies.

MORE STUFF:

I'm a Certified Health Coach
And Personal Trainer.
I have gained 100 lbs. I have lost 100 lbs.
I moved to my dream town
and hike almost daily.
I have a new puppy named Kona.
I am learning to surf.
I have a 20 min morning Superpower Practice.
I can make fire by rubbing sticks together.
I said no to Cancer. This is my first book.

TAKE IT TO THE NEXT LEVEL

LET'S WORK TOGETHER

www.gritstrong.com

CONNECT W/ ME

www.gritstrong.com

www.facebook.com/gritstrong

www.scoop.it/u/natalie-galyon

www.pinterest.com/GRITSTRONG

www.instagram.com/gritphotos

www.youtube.com/nataliegalyon

Please get in touch for health coaching, online fitness training, speaking events, and online classes.

Who made the world? Who made the swan, and the black bear? Who made the grasshopper? This grasshopper, I mean- the one who has flung herself out of the grass, the one who is eating sugar out of my hand, who is moving her jaws back and forth instead of up and down- who is gazing around with her enormous and complicated eyes. Now she lifts her pale forearms and thoroughly washes her face. Now she snaps her wings open, and floats away. I don't know exactly what a prayer is. I do know how to pay attention, how to fall down into the grass, how to kneel down in the grass, how to be idle and blessed, how to stroll through the fields, which is what I have been doing all day. **Tell me, what else should I have done?** Doesn't everything die at last, and too soon? **Tell me, what is it you plan to do with your one wild and precious life?**
- Mary Oliver